Raising Awareness for the Prevention of Workplace Violence, Bullying, and Active Shooter Training in Healthcare

An Instructional Guide on Awareness, Prevention of Violence, Bullying and Active Shooter Issues in the Workplace

by Zack Thomas, RN

Contents

Introduction

The naïve among us have a very bright outlook on how the healthcare industry functions. They consider it to be a noble profession where one saves lives, and it certainly is. However, few people understand the risks that come along the way, and even fewer are prepared for the challenges.

My name is Zack Thomas, and I'm here to shed light on a largely overlooked aspect of working in healthcare — violence, bullying, and active shooter situations, particularly as they affect the nursing staff.

As a registered nurse (RN) with years of experience in healthcare, I can tell you there exists a gap that many in healthcare feel — though hospitals aim to provide compassionate care, support for staff safety can sometimes fall short. Those affected by these shortcomings might label the system as uncaring; however, from my experience as an emergency room nurse and a house supervisor and having witnessed firsthand the violence healthcare workers endure, I can say with confidence that there are ways to bridge this gap with training and awareness. This is why I founded Empirical Safety Training. The goal of my company is to partner with hospitals, nursing facilities, and psychiatric centers to provide comprehensive training on violence prevention, ensuring compliance with California's AB508 and SB1299 state laws. These laws, enforced by the California Division of Occupational Safety and Health (OSHA), mandate that all healthcare facilities implement active violence prevention training programs for their employees and contractors. These trainings are not optional — they must be conducted annually.

For the past 25 years, I've practiced and trained in various forms of martial arts, and this, combined with my medical experience, laid the foundation for my company. I am also an active contributing member of the International Association of Healthcare Safety and Security (IAHSS) and a registered provider with the California Board of Registered Nursing, allowing me to offer students the Continuing Education Units (CEUs) credits that they need to fulfill their professional requirements.

But why focus on nursing staff, in particular? The reason is simple: many new nurses enter the industry without being aware of the bullying and outright violence they may encounter. Resources to help them get through these situations are often scarce, and many have no idea how to respond.

It's time for a change, and that change starts with active measures to make the profession safer, more supportive, and more self-aware. I feel it is my moral and civic duty to shine a light on this critical issue within the healthcare industry.

As things currently stand, there is already a shortage of approximately 36,000 licensed nurses in California[1] — a problem made worse by workplace violence and bullying. The statistics speak for themselves. According to a survey[2]:

- In 2023, 43.4% of nurses have reported incidents of workplace violence

[1] https://sd31.senate.ca.gov/news/2024-05-22-sacramento-bee-california-facing-nursing-shortage-community-colleges-might-be

[2] Friese, C. R., Medvec, B. R., Marriott, D. J., Khadr, L., Wade, M. G., Riba, M., & Titler, M. G. (2024). Nurse-reported workplace violent events: Results from a repeated statewide survey. Nursing Outlook, 72(5), 102265. https://doi.org/10.1016/j.outlook.2024.102265

- 55.3% of nurses have reported a violent incident to their employer
- Employer response was less than half the time
- In the reported incidents, the sources of violence were as follows:
  - 54.5% - patients
  - 26.1% - peers
  - 18.8% - visitors
- The most common instances of workplace violence were linked to:
  - Poor work conditions
  - Inadequate staffing
  - Younger age

These statistics reveal a systemic issue. Even when incidents of workplace violence are reported, employers often fail to take notice or action. More concerning is that a significant portion of violence comes from peers, highlighting the urgent need for awareness and change. This book is an effort to drive that change.

I will guide you through an in-depth exploration of violence and bullying in the healthcare industry, as well as discuss practical, proactive measures to address and eliminate these issues. We must work together to combat the nursing shortage, and to do so, we will focus on strategies for building healthy teamwork, embracing the industry's natural and cultural diversity, improving communication, fostering emotional intelligence, and creating greater self-awareness.

Nursing Code of Ethics and Workplace Violence

Just like doctors have to take a Hippocratic oath, nurses must also adhere to a code of ethics.

The Code of Ethics for Nursing is an essential guide for professional conduct in the field of nursing. It outlines the ethical responsibilities nurses have toward their patients, colleagues, and the public, ensuring they maintain high standards of care and professionalism. The significance of the code lies in its ability to protect the integrity of the nursing profession, promote patient well-being, and create respectful and supportive work environments.

While the code of ethics has several provisions, one of the most important provisions in the code is 1.5 - **Relationships with Colleagues and Others**, which states:

> *"The nurse creates an ethical environment and culture of civility and kindness, treating colleagues, co-workers, employees, students, and others with dignity and respect. This standard of conduct includes an affirmative duty to act to prevent harm. Disregard for the effects of one's actions on others, bullying, harassment, intimidation, manipulation, threats, or violence are always morally unacceptable behaviors."[3]*

This particular provision clearly explains the responsibility of nurses to maintain a professional and respectful

---

[3] https://www.nursingworld.org/practice-policy/nursing-excellence/ethics/code-of-ethics-for-nurses/

environment while actively preventing harm to others. Unfortunately, despite this clear ethical guideline, not all nurses adhere to it, leading to bullying and workplace violence, especially against travel and registry nurses, who are more vulnerable due to their temporary status.

But how exactly are violence and bullying carried out in the field? Let's find out.

Violence

Violence is defined as any physical activity that leads to the bodily assault of a person. It can also cause mental and emotional harm. Such actions are done with the intent to hurt someone.

Violence is broadly characterized in the following manner:

- **Verbal Abuse:** This includes all threatening behavior, threats, or casual comments made, like expressing the intention to hurt or harm someone. It can also include moments of physical intimidation, either through threatening body language, the destruction of property, or personal belongings to instill fear.
- **Physical Abuse:** Actions of physical abuse that lead to bodily harm are known as physical abuse. These actions are legally classified as assault. Assault can be of various types, based on:
  - Whether a weapon was used (aggravated assault)
  - The harm was sexual (sexual assault)
  - If a severe bodily injury occurred (aggravated assault)
  - Murder (First degree, second-degree, etc.)

Under Senate Bill 1299, workplace violence is identified as all actions that cause harm to another person. It can be perpetrated by a patient, their relatives, or even co-workers. Additionally, all acts of violence or aggression are punishable by law.

Types of Violence in Healthcare

Most people assume that violence is generally of two types – it's either physical or verbal. According to the *Emergency Care Research Institute* (ECRI), that is not true. In reality, there are four main types of violence, especially in the healthcare industry.[4]

However, there is one additional type of violence that is not included in the ECRI's list. Luckily, we're going to be discussing this extra type here in addition to the four mentioned above.

Type 1: Criminal Intent

Violence with criminal intent is the first type of workplace violence we're going to look at. Criminal intent is classified in the following manner:

- It occurs in scenarios where the perpetrator has no direct connection or relationship with the hospital or the employees who are present at a hospital or a clinic.
- It's usually done for the sake of the resources that are found in hospitals, such as medication, medical equipment, money, etc.
- This type of violence is committed by thieves, mobsters, drug addicts, or anyone else who is just looking to loot the resources present at hospitals.
- This violence is mostly physical, involves the use of weapons, and can result in people getting assaulted indiscriminately.

---

[4] https://www.ecri.org/components/HRC/Pages/SafSec3.aspx

- This can happen inside the hospital or outside, in the parking lot, but usually, they pick instances when there will be fewer people to witness the violence.
- Sometimes, this type of violence might not occur on the hospital premises. For example, a healthcare worker might get mugged while they are visiting someone's home for in-house duties, which can cause a lot of bodily harm to them.
- Violence with criminal intent is rare on hospital grounds and premises as compared to other types of violence.

Type 2: Customer/Client
The second type of workplace violence is probably the most common one that occurs in a hospital. Customer client violence is classified on the following details:

- It relates to the relationship between the customer or client and a healthcare worker. The client/customer in this scenario includes the patient, their family members, and any visitors.
- Any or all of these people could become verbally or physically abusive towards registered nurses.
- The most common occurrence is verbal abuse, but heated arguments have resulted in people's physical abuse.
- Patients, visitors, and their family members have been known to resort to hitting, pushing, punching, or hurting the nurses that they are interacting with.
- Physical violence that comes directly from patients is not very common among mentally fit clients, but you can still expect verbal abuse.
- Physical violence is most likely to occur either during psychiatric treatment or in waiting rooms.

- Often, the patient may need to be physically restrained to stop them from harming not only others but themselves as well.

Type 3: Worker on Worker (Lateral Violence)

The third type of violence is inflicted by healthcare workers on other healthcare workers. It can be classified on the following basis:

- The co-workers can either be people in the same office and designation or people who work in a higher or lower position than that person.
- It is also known as *horizontal* or *lateral violence* since it happens between co-workers.
- This may start either covertly or overtly with bullying that can turn into emotional and verbal abuse. An example of this can be seen in the use of offensive speech, playing off the use of derogatory words by calling it a joke, humiliating another employee in public by yelling at them, being unfair to another employee, etc.
- This type of violence can escalate if no active measures are taken.
- It can stop being emotionally or verbally abusive and move to become physically abusive.
- This is also something that starts very slowly. It could be slight shoves or pushes, light grabbing of the arm, pulling off the hair, and getting into one's personal space.
- As the aggressor bends the personal boundaries of the other person, they can inflict more verbal or physical abuse on the person.

- This type of violence is extremely dangerous as it can slowly lead the way to serious physical or sexual assault like rape or murder.
- Worker-on-worker violence is more common in a hierarchal chain as it naturally makes it very easy to control or manipulate someone, especially when someone is aware that they belong to a position that is below someone.

Type 4: Personal Relationships
The fourth type of workplace violence is not related to the workplace – it just occurs there. It can be classified as the following:

- It relates to scenarios where an employee or worker may be in a personal relationship with someone who shows up to their workplace to abuse them.
- These scenarios usually involve acts of violence that are caused by abusive partners.
- Violence of this nature can get serious quickly since it is a form of emotional abuse that, if allowed to, can quickly devolve into physical abuse, too.
- It's usually an effort by the abuser to humiliate and embarrass their victim so much that there's no place left that will accept the person. They will have no choice but to return to the abuser.
- The abuser may use covert tactics, such as intimidation stalking, that slowly spill into verbal and physical harassment and turn into beatings, shootings, or stabbings.
- They might only target one person, or they might even threaten others, including the patients and co-workers of their victims.

The deadly outcomes of this type of violence have been seen in hospitals all over. Just in 2018, a doctor named Dr. Tamara O'Neal was gunned down in an active shooter situation by a man named Juan Lopez. The reason for the killing was apparently over a *"broken engagement"* between the shooter and the doctor.[5]

But it's not always women who are the victim. These acts of violence are carried out against men by women or people of the same gender, too. Reasons for this can range from lust, envy, and revenge to suspicions of cheating, stalking, or just raw resentment. This type of workplace violence may not be as common, but when it occurs, it can have harmful consequences.

Type 5: Ideological Violence
This last form of violence is known as ideological violence. It is identified based on the following:

- This is caused by people who use violence to achieve some form of a personal, sociopolitical goal.
- This type of violence also comes under the umbrella of terrorism because a terrorist is a person who performs terrible acts that cause harm or shock society to promote their group's agenda.
- Personal desires or grudges rarely motivate this form of violence.
- It's always the ideology and belief system of the person or group that leads to this course of action.
- In most cases of ideological violence, the person who commits the act doesn't work alone. The assailant or

---

[5]https://www.chicagotribune.com/2018/11/20/chicago-hospital-shooting-young-cop-doctor-pharmacy-resident-and-gunman-die-in-mercy-hospital-attack-2/

the terrorist is usually part of a group that has a particular belief system and plan for the attack.

- They will usually believe that this act will help them get closer to achieving their goal.
- These terrorist acts also help obscure terrorist groups gain attention and recognition among the public. This helps them establish a more powerful position in the eyes of the public.
- Another reason is that hospitals are full of the most vulnerable and weak, and terrorists can get more media attention and a prompt response from authorities if they perform a violent act there.
- Hospitals can be vulnerable to such attacks and may also have a high amount of hostages.
- In healthcare, this form of violence may vary because each case can be different.

Self Awareness

Empirical Safety Training

What is Self-Awareness?

Self-Awareness is Having a Clear Perception of Your Personality

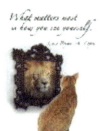

This includes your strengths, weaknesses, thoughts, beliefs, motivations, and emotions.

Self-awareness allows you to understand other people, how they perceive you, your attitude and your responses to them in the moment.

Notes:_____
_____
_____
_____
_____
_____
_____
_____
_____
_____

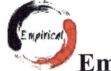 **Empirical Safety Training**

Self-Awareness Risk Factors

- ❖ Working Directly with Volatile People
  - ▪ If they are currently under the influence of drugs
  - ▪ History of violence related to psychotic diagnosis
  - ▪ Disgruntle family members
- ❖ Transporting Patients
- ❖ Long Waits for Service
- ❖ Overcrowded, Uncomfortable Waiting Rooms
- ❖ Working Alone

Elevated Levels of Stress

- ❖ Lack of staff training and policies for preventing and managing crises with potentially volatile patients
- ❖ Lack of team support
- ❖ Avoid playing favoritism with staff (Supervisors/Management)
- ❖ Poorly lit corridors, rooms, parking lots, and other areas (notify security if areas are not well-lit)
- ❖ Workplace Bullying (See next section)

Notes:_____

_____

_____

_____

_____

_____

_____

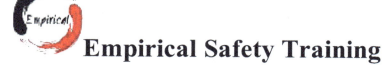

Empirical Safety Training

Self-Awareness   Personal   Empowerment
Therapeutic Techniques

- ❖ **Modifying Interactions**
    - ✓ **Take a Break**
    - ✓ **Remove Yourself From the Situation**
- ❖ **Restructuring**
    - ✓ **Boundary Setting**
    - ✓ **Challenge Unproductive Assumptions**
    - ✓ **Use Intensity to Cause Change (Do Not Give Up)**
    - ✓ **Promote Competency**
    - ✓ **Take Responsibility for Yourself and Your Own Actions**
    - ✓ **Encourage Co-Workers to be Responsible for Themselves and Their Actions**

Notes:_____

_____

_____

_____

_____

_____

_____

_____

_____

_____

_____

_____

_____

The Culture of Bullying

According to the American Nurses Association, bullying is defined as *repeated, unwanted, harmful actions intended to humiliate, offend, and cause distress in the recipient.*[6]

Bullying remains a major issue in schools across the U.S., affecting millions of children each year. According to the National Center for Educational Statistics, about 19% of students ages 12-18 experience bullying in some form.[7]

The impact can be devastating, causing the ones impacted to suffer from anxiety, depression, and a lack of self-worth. In severe cases, bullying has led to tragic outcomes such as school shootings. Children who are bullied are more likely to see a drop in their grades, struggle to form relationships, and may even develop long-term mental health issues.

According to a report released by the U.S. Secret Service National Threat Assessment Center, almost 80% of the perpetrators involved in school shootings were subject to bullying. [8] But that's not all. In many cases, students who experience bullying are more likely to consider or attempt suicide than their peers.

When children are bullied, parents often step in by contacting school authorities, arranging meetings with teachers, or even pulling their children from the environment altogether to ensure their safety. The focus is on protecting

---

[6] https://www.nursingworld.org/practice-policy/work-environment/end-nurse-abuse/
[7] https://nces.ed.gov/fastfacts/display.asp?id=719
[8]https://www.k12dive.com/news/bullying-school-shootings-prevention/704206/#

the child and finding solutions to the problem. However, what happens when adults experience bullying in the workplace? Unfortunately, bullying doesn't stop at the classroom door. It follows many into adulthood, impacting their jobs, well-being, and daily lives.

Bullying in the Nursing Field

The problem with bullying in the nursing field begins taking root at an early stage. According to a study published in Nursing Administration Quarterly, almost 78% of students face bullying during nursing school, which signifies that the problem starts way before a person can step into the professional world. More concerning is the fact that 34% of nurses end up leaving or consider leaving the profession entirely because of bullying.[9]

While bullying comes under the category of worker-on-worker violence, as mentioned in the previous section, due to its prevalence in nursing, it is important to discuss it separately.

A well-known phrase in nursing, "Nurses eat their young," highlights the harsh reality many new nurses face when entering the profession. Older or more experienced nurses sometimes treat younger colleagues harshly, creating a toxic work environment. Instead of learning from their past experiences, such nurses repeat the cycle of bullying that they themselves may have faced at some point in their careers. This behavior not only affects the mental and emotional health of travel and registry nurses but also compromises patient care.

---

[9] Edmonson, C., & Zelonka, C. (2019). Our Own Worst Enemies: The Nurse Bullying Epidemic. Nursing administration quarterly, 43(3), 274–279. https://doi.org/10.1097/NAQ.0000000000000353

Nurses are already stressed out due to the excessive workload and the fact that they are dealing with patients of all kinds. It certainly isn't a walk in the park, and bullying doesn't make the job any easier. Worse yet, workplace bullying has contributed to active shooter incidents and violent outbursts in the past. It just goes to show the intense pressure and frustration that can build in such hostile environments.

Bullying in healthcare also contradicts the very values we teach our children. We tell kids to stand up against bullies and to treat others with respect and kindness. Yet, in some hospitals, bullying is not only tolerated but perpetuated by those in leadership roles. This hypocrisy sends a mixed message to the next generation and creates a dangerous cycle where violence and harassment become normalized.

It is only natural to have co-workers you don't get along with. But that doesn't mean you need to harass them at work. There are far too many active shooter cases in today's society to ignore. We need to treat people and co-workers who work just as hard as everyone else with kindness and compassion. It is time to raise awareness and educate others about anti-bullying practices.

That said, let's explore the different types of bullying in the healthcare industry.

Overt Bullying
Overt bullying refers to bullying that is obvious and easy to identify. It's more direct and can include actions like belittling a colleague by harshly criticizing their work, especially in front of others, which undermines their confidence.

Minimizing a fellow nurse's struggles by telling them to "suck it up" is another common form of overt bullying, dismissing their concerns rather than offering support. Name-calling, such as labeling someone a "bad nurse" or yelling to intimidate or scare them, also falls into this category.

In more extreme cases, overt bullying may even involve physical aggression, like pushing or shoving or preventing someone from moving freely by blocking their way. These actions are openly aggressive and clearly damaging to the work environment.

Covert Bullying
Covert bullying is more subtle but can be equally harmful. It involves actions that are less noticeable but still intended to hurt or isolate a person. For instance, ostracizing a colleague, which involves purposely excluding them from conversations or group activities, can damage morale and make the victim feel isolated. Gossiping or spreading rumors about another nurse can also contribute to a toxic work culture and harm the reputation of the person being targeted. Another example of covert bullying is ignoring a fellow nurse's calls for help during a difficult task. This passive form of bullying leaves the nurse vulnerable, forcing them to manage dangerous situations alone or wait for help, delaying care and increasing stress.

The Impact of Bullying on Patient Care
Nurse bullying has a serious impact on the quality of patient care. When nurses are subjected to hostile behavior, it creates a tense and stressful work environment, which can hinder their ability to focus on providing the best possible care. The emotional toll of being bullied may cause nurses to feel isolated, anxious, or insecure, leading to increased

mental fatigue and decreased job satisfaction. This can translate into less attentiveness to patient needs, slower response times, and lower overall performance.

The stress and anxiety brought on by bullying can also impair a nurse's ability to think clearly and make sound decisions. Ultimately, it leads to treatment errors, mistakes in administering medications, or failure to adhere to important protocols. In high-pressure situations, where quick and accurate decision-making is required, a bullied nurse may struggle to remain calm and focused. Furthermore, the fear of being targeted or ridiculed by colleagues may cause nurses to hesitate before asking for help, which leads to errors that could have been avoided.

When communication between healthcare professionals breaks down due to bullying, it directly affects the level of care patients receive. Nurses may be reluctant to report changes in a patient's condition out of fear of backlash or further bullying from colleagues. The delay in communication can result in slower interventions, delayed treatments, and longer recovery times. In the most serious cases, it may even lead to patient mortality.

In addition, the quality of the nurse-patient relationship is often undermined when bullying is present. A nurse who is stressed or emotionally drained may appear distracted, unengaged, or irritable when interacting with patients. As a result, patients may feel neglected, uncared for, or dissatisfied with the care they receive, which damages trust in the healthcare system as a whole.

A study published in Human Resources for Health identified several significant themes that impact patient care due to bullying in healthcare, including patient falls, errors in treatment or medication, delayed care, adverse events or patient mortality, impaired thinking or concentration, inhibited communication, and lowered patient satisfaction or an increase in patient complaints.[10] These findings highlight the severe consequences of bullying in healthcare environments.

The Impact of Bullying on Nurses

Besides patient care, bullying in the workplace also has a significant effect on the well-being of nurses. Being repeatedly subjected to hostile or undermining behavior can lead to emotional exhaustion, anxiety, and depression.

With time, these feelings can erode a nurse's confidence and sense of self-worth, causing them to question their professional abilities. The constant stress is enough to make it difficult to maintain focus or stay motivated. Ultimately, it leads to disengagement from the work environment.

The emotional strain caused by bullying can also affect physical health. Nurses who experience bullying often report chronic stress-related conditions, such as headaches, fatigue, and gastrointestinal issues. These physical symptoms, coupled with emotional distress, make it hard for nurses to stay fully present at work. The continuous tension disrupts sleep patterns and contributes to burnout, making it increasingly difficult for them to recover between shifts.

In addition to personal health deterioration, nurses who face bullying often struggle to maintain positive relationships with colleagues. They may feel isolated or fearful of

---

[10]Al Omar, M., Salam, M. & Al-Surimi, K. Workplace bullying and its impact on the quality of healthcare and patient safety. Hum Resour Health 17, 89 (2019). https://doi.org/10.1186/s12960-019-0433-x

speaking up, which limits their ability to communicate openly with the team.

The long-term effects of bullying in the nursing profession are concerning, as they lead to higher turnover rates. Nurses who experience consistent bullying may decide to leave the profession altogether, taking with them valuable experience and expertise. The nurse shortage already exists, so when more nurses leave, it creates additional pressure on the remaining staff members.

According to a study published in the Western Journal of Nursing Research, nurses who are bullied at work experience poorer physical and mental health, which lowers their overall quality of life. The decline in well-being also interferes with their ability to provide safe, effective patient care, further illuminating the serious consequences of bullying within healthcare settings.[11]

---

[11] Sauer, Penny A, and Thomas P McCoy. "Nurse Bullying: Impact on Nurses' Health." Western journal of nursing research vol. 39,12 (2017): 1533-1546. doi:10.1177/0193945916681278

How to Catch a Covert Bully

We spoke of overt and covert forms of bullying in the previous chapter. While overt bullying is obvious, in healthcare settings, nurses are more likely to face covert or subtle forms of bullying.

Once you recognize you are being bullied, it is essential to take action. But how exactly can you do that? Here are three ways to catch a covert bully:

Step 1: Join Forces

When law enforcement agents are tasked with apprehending a dangerous criminal, their first step is to collaborate across agencies. The FBI, local police, and any other relevant parties come together as a single unit. They share every piece of evidence and lead and pool their resources to ensure the criminal is caught. Similarly, in the healthcare field, nurses should adopt a collaborative approach when facing covert bullying.

If a nurse finds themselves dealing with a difficult charge nurse, seeking help is essential. Nurses should turn to the human resources department, supervisors, and even directors to gather support. Each of these resources can provide a different perspective and may have the authority to address the problem directly.

However, before taking action, make sure to thoroughly review hospital policies and the code of conduct. It will help identify specific violations that the charge nurse may be committing. Look for a pattern of bullying behavior, lack of fairness, or failure to comply with ethical standards. Understanding the hospital's policies will provide a clear direction for addressing the issue. These guidelines are the evidence that can be used to make a formal complaint or take steps toward resolution.

Nurses should also document their own experiences and interactions with the charge nurse in question. This will help build a case if there's a need to escalate the situation. Combining this documentation with insights from hospital policies creates a strong foundation for addressing covert bullying.

Step 2: Confront the Bully

To continue with the law enforcement example, when they have enough evidence leading to a suspect, they bring them in for questioning. Confronting a covert bully in healthcare requires directly communicating with them. Once you've gathered enough evidence or noticed repeated patterns of negative behavior, it's important to address the issue head-on. Confronting the bully, whether they are a peer or a charge nurse, will bring attention to the problem and potentially put an end to the toxic behavior.

It is important to stay calm and professional when you approach the bully. Tell them straight out that their behavior is compromising patient care and disrupting the work environment. Be specific about the actions you've observed. It could range from undermining colleagues and fostering an unfair atmosphere to directly violating hospital policies. Make it clear that this behavior is not only affecting morale but could also be putting patient safety at risk.

It's important to state your expectations clearly. Explain exactly how you want them to change their behavior. For instance, if the bully is a charge nurse who is unfairly distributing assignments or targeting specific staff members, let them know that their actions are being observed and will not be tolerated. Setting clear expectations creates accountability, even when addressing someone in a leadership role.

Make sure to inform them that continued violations will lead to consequences. Make it known that if the bullying behavior does not stop, you will escalate the issue through the appropriate channels.

Step 3: Build a Case

If your warning doesn't change the bully's behavior, it's time to move to the final step — building a case. Start documenting every instance of inappropriate behavior. Whether the documentation comes from your own experiences or from colleagues, collect everything relevant. This could include reports of mistreatment, incidents of policy violations, or other actions that have been witnessed. It doesn't matter if the reports are anonymous or signed — what matters is building a comprehensive record.

This process may take some time but don't get discouraged. Much like a jury decides a case based on the weight of the evidence, HR or hospital administration will make decisions based on the patterns and facts you present. The stronger and more detailed your case, the harder it will be for the bully to defend their actions.

Once you've built a solid case, the goal should be to ensure that the charge nurse or bully is removed from their position of power. This could mean requesting their removal from leadership roles or recommending that they no longer manage a team. If they are leading any committees, push for their removal from those positions as well. The objective is to make sure they no longer hold influence over others in the workplace.

Wrapping up, I would like to acknowledge Renee Thompson, CEO and Founder of the Healthy Workforce Institute, for her dedication to helping healthcare leaders address bullying and incivility in their organizations. Her expertise and resources are invaluable for anyone seeking to create healthier workplace cultures.

Developing an Anti-Bullying Workplace Policy

Implementing an anti-bullying policy in the workplace establishes a clear expectation for respectful and professional behavior among employees. In healthcare, the absence of such a policy allows harmful behaviors to persist. This not only affects morale but can also lead to unfair practices, which have the potential to damage a nurse's career without valid justification.

Below is a bullying mitigation policy developed by Empirical Safety Training:

Entity(s): Empirical Safety Training Policy: Anti-Workplace Bully Prevention

Purpose: The purpose of this policy is to establish guidelines dealing with toxic workplace bully from coworkers and peers, which undermines everyone's safety:

Bullying is an intentional, unwanted, aggressive, repetitive behavior that involves real or perceived power imbalance that hurts, harms, and humiliates an individual. Either physically or emotionally, causing a toxic environment.

Objectives: The policy aims to improve the quality of services to our patients, promoting an atmosphere of civility and teamwork with respect for others with whom we come in contact. The workplace has zero tolerance for workplace bullying.

Strategies to Achieve Objectives: Strategies to improve the quality of the workplace include:

- Self-awareness
- Fostering a culture of continuous civility
- Respect of others
- Self-control
- Abiding by rules
- Honesty
- Compassion
- Offer help
- Politeness

Specific Actions to be Taken: This policy recommends the following actions:

- Remain Calm
- Identify the source
- Approach the individual when the timing is right
- Be polite
- Take a breath
- Inform the individual of the situation and how it made you feel
- Listen for readback if receptive
- Offer solutions to move forward. If not, notify your chain of command

Desired Outcomes of Specific Actions: The desired outcomes of this policy are as follows:

- Every employee should be free of harassing behaviors.

Performance Indicators:

- Increase civility
- Increase teamwork support
- Increase humility

- Increase productivity
- Decrease liability cost
- Decrease turnover rate

The success of this policy may be measured in terms of better management of risk associated with workplace bullying.

Management plans and day-to-day operational rules should cover aspects of adherence to the zero workplace bullying policy.

Root Cause Analysis:

- Non-bias
- Take every complaint seriously
- Investigate properly
- Medication
- Notify employees according to the hospital policy
- Only facts
- Offer solutions
- EAP

This policy should be reviewed annually. The Review Process should include an examination of the performance indicators. Consultation with members of the committee and discussion forum involving the Management Committee and Risk Management Professionals.

Workplace Violence in American Healthcare

Statistics show nearly 2 million Americans face incidents of workplace violence each year. Out of these 2 million, almost 78% of instances of workplace violence are experienced by healthcare workers. [12]

But, the problem is out of all healthcare workers; nurses are more likely to face instances of workplace violence. While in many cases, the violence is not physical, it still takes a toll on the nurse's mental health, as explained previously.

In 2022, a tragic incident at Methodist Dallas Medical Center highlighted the dangers healthcare workers face. Nestor Hernandez, a man who had been paroled after serving time for robbery, is now charged with capital murder. Hernandez was visiting his girlfriend in the hospital after she gave birth when he accused her of cheating and violently attacked her. He then shot and killed two hospital workers — Jaqueline Pokuaa, a nurse, and Katie Flowers, a social worker — before being shot and detained by police. [13]

This heartbreaking incident is just one example of the violence that healthcare workers, especially nurses, are exposed to. According to statistics from the U.S. Bureau of Labor Statistics, during the pandemic, violence in the workplace has risen, and nurses are three times more likely to face this danger than people in other jobs.

---

[12] https://wifitalents.com/statistic/work-place-violence/
[13] https://abcnews.go.com/US/dead-gunman-opens-fire-dallas-hospital-officials/story?id=91917260

Healthcare workers, whose main goal is to help and care for others, should never have to fear for their safety at work. The rising risk to their well-being highlights the need for stronger protections.

According to the National Nurse United (NUU), 8 out of 10 nurses have experienced an incident of workplace violence in their career. But what's even more concerning is the fact only 29.5% of employers have the means to mitigate instances of violence. [14]

Given the history of workplace violence in healthcare, it is the responsibility of all employers to have mitigation teams or dedicated staff that can control instances of violence before they end up claiming more lives.

---

[14] https://www.nationalnursesunited.org/press/nnu-report-shows-increased-rates-of-workplace-violence-experienced-by-nurses

The Assembly Bill 508

The history of violent incidents in hospitals and healthcare facilities has been known for a long time, but a major event in 1993 pushed authorities to take more serious action.

That year, a tragic shooting occurred at the Los Angeles County-USC Medical Center when a disgruntled patient, Damacio Torres, targeted medical staff in a terrifying act of violence. Torres, who had been receiving medical treatment for over a decade, reportedly believed the care he was given was substandard. His frustration escalated, leading him to shoot two doctors and a nurse in the hospital's emergency room.

The incident unfolded in a walk-in clinic that typically saw around 300 patients a day for minor injuries and ailments. As Torres took hostages for five hours, the hospital staff faced an unimaginable situation. Police responded quickly, and non-essential workers on the first floor of the massive 2,045-bed hospital were evacuated as a safety measure. Meanwhile, new patients were diverted to other hospitals. Torres eventually surrendered, but the damage was done — both physically and emotionally to the victims and to the sense of security in healthcare environments.

This tragic event served as a wake-up call, prompting California lawmakers to act. In the wake of the shooting, Assembly Bill 508 (AB508) was passed. The bill was created to provide better protection for healthcare workers and strengthen measures to prevent violence in hospitals.

AB 508

The Assembly Bill (AB) 508 made it mandatory for all hospital healthcare employees to receive the appropriate training in different emergency scenarios.

A hospital, nursing home, or nursing facility is legally obligated to teach healthcare workers about how to handle verbal abuse and physical assault. Under this bill, healthcare workers need to be made aware of and trained to know exactly what to do if they are in danger at their jobs.

According to Assembly Bill 508, all hospital employees and personnel must report any incidents of battery or assault to their local enforcement agencies within 72 hours. Their report will then be investigated, and the perpetrators can face jail time, penalties, or both.

Through this bill, more healthcare employees are encouraged to learn how to de-escalate high-risk situations and how to protect themselves. This training is useful not just for nurses but also for all hospital personnel, including:

- Physicians
- Paramedics
- Social workers
- Technicians
- Therapists and
- The security guards

The AB 508 bill made it compulsory for hospitals to actively assess any potential threats to the safety of their healthcare workers. Hospitals have to test their current security measures and safety plans regularly. This is done to evaluate whether a hospital is prepared for the different kinds of potentially violent situations that can occur on its premises.

All hospitals are required to have detailed emergency plans to effectively tackle identified violent situations, especially if they pose a risk to the safety of their staff and personnel.

Mandatory Training as Defined by the AB 508

According to AB 508, the following are some critical areas that the workplace violence training program should focus on:

- A healthcare worker must be taught the right measures to take for general and personal safety. They should know how to keep themselves safe in harmful situations in the workplace.
- Healthcare workers are educated on the assault and crisis cycle and how to deal with it at the workplace.
- Healthcare workers are taught how to communicate with patients who have histories of violence. This allows them to approach severe or violent patients with appropriate caution. They know how to speak to such patients and can assess when a conversation is:
  o Turning into a heated argument
  o Could devolve into a violent situation
  o Become an active shooter situation
  o Cause an incident that puts lives at risk.
- Healthcare workers will learn to identify the common characteristics of violent patients. This knowledge allows healthcare workers to apply appropriate precautions when dealing with violent patients. They also learn about potential triggers and the patient's anger response.
- Healthcare workers will learn proper verbal and physical techniques and how to deal with violent patients or co-workers.

- Healthcare workers learn to use maneuvers to save themselves from a violent attacker. They can develop evasive strategies to escape from or restrain violent people. This is an important skill to possess, especially when you need to keep an attacker in control while you wait for help to arrive.
- Healthcare workers have to learn about medications or chemicals they can use to restrain an attacker. Healthcare workers will need to practice administering medication that can successfully disable an attacker and stop them from causing further harm.
- Lastly, healthcare workers need to learn about the resources at their disposal if they are involved in a violent incident. They need to be aware of reporting requirements, possible employee assistance programs, and other resources available for healthcare workers who have experienced violent situations.

It's easy to see that AB 508 is designed to make hospitals take active measures to improve the work environment and the lives of healthcare professionals in the U.S.

Understanding Instances of Assault at Work

Apart from understanding the types of violence discussed previously, you also need to understand the different types of assault as per AB 508. Most people generally believe that physical abuse is a form of abuse only. However, when one has to report it, they will see that physical abuse is identified differently. You need to be aware of this, especially if you want to report the issue accurately.

In the law, physical abuse is defined as assault. Assault is when a person inflicts physical harm on another person. It also includes instances where a person touches someone without their consent. Assault is a crime, so the perpetrator will have to answer to the law for their actions.

To charge someone with assault, the victim will have to make a case and provide evidence to prove that the assault occurred. Assault can occur in many different spaces, including the workplace and even in the home.

Additionally, assault is not a blanket term. Based on the kind of physical action and harm, there are different kinds of assault. The following are the ones that you should know about:

Simple Assault
This type of assault happens without the use of any weapons. The injuries caused by these can be minor.

Physical Assault (Battery)
This is also known as a battery. This type of assault can be further understood and identified based on the following factors:

- This form of assault occurs when a perpetrator applies physical force to another person without their consent.
- This occurs without a weapon, and injuries from this form of assault are usually minimal.
- This can include actions such as merely blocking another person's path, pushing, shoving, or hitting someone.
- It can also be considered as intent to assault if someone is threatening you while visibly holding anything that can be used as a weapon.
- The weapon can be any sharp or heavy object, a tool, a container of dangerous chemicals, or a gun.

- It will be considered assault even if the perpetrator attempts to use an object that doesn't qualify as a weapon, such as throwing a pen at someone's face.

Aggravated Assault

This type of assault can be further understood and identified based on the following factors:

- If serious bodily harm occurs from an assault, it will be classified as aggravated assault.
- Aggravated assault is when severe bodily harm occurs with or without the use of a weapon.
- Bodily harm in this category includes all actions that can cut, maim, wound, bruise, disfigure, or pose a risk to the victim's life.
- Usually, the nature of the injuries will also show that a weapon was used.
- Aggravated assault is seen as a criminal crime, which means that this action is punishable by jail time.
- Victims must report any crimes of aggravated assault to put the person behind bars.

Sexual Assault

This type of assault can be further understood and identified based on the following factors:

- This form of assault occurs when a person forces someone to engage in sexual activity without their consent.
- Sexual assault is not the same as sexual harassment.
- Sexual harassment encompasses verbal and minor physical acts that are sexually inappropriate without someone's consent.
- When the harassment starts to include physical acts of violence where a person is raped or coerced with

threats into sexual activity, it is known as sexual assault.
- The victim usually fears for his/her life in this scenario.

It is unfortunate that in healthcare, it is common for a lot of female nurses to be the victims of sexual assault or sexual harassment by their co-workers and bosses and, in rare cases, their patients.

Aggravated Sexual Assault
- This type of assault can be further understood and identified based on the following factors:
- Aggravated sexual assault is when a person inflicts severe bodily harm on another person while forcing them to engage in sexual activity.
- This bodily harm includes wounding, maiming, disfiguring, or disabling a victim.
- It can be committed with a weapon to threaten the victim or inflict bodily harm to make the victim cooperative.
- The crime can also be aided and abetted by another person.
- Anyone who experiences aggravated sexual assault is requested to report it.
- Many victims choose to remain silent, but that often means that the abuser gets to walk free.
- If you do choose to speak up, you will get all the help you need, starting with the medical staff that helps you.

By understanding these forms of assault, you can easily ensure that you or anyone else you know is aware of how to identify the physical abuse they suffered.

The Senate Bill 1299

Another bill for health care professionals is the Senate Bill 1299 (SB 1299). This was passed in 2014 and made it mandatory for all hospitals to follow the safety and security standards as defined by the *Division of Occupational Safety and Health (DOSH)* or the *Occupational Safety and Health Standards Board (OSHA)*. The bill is designed to be an effective workplace violence prevention plan.

It is based on the definition that OSHA uses to identify workplace violence. According to OSHA, the definition of workplace violence is *"Any act or threat of physical violence, harassment, intimidation, or other threatening disruptive behavior that occurs at the worksite. It ranges from threats and verbal abuse to physical assaults and even homicide."*[15]

This definition is so apt that the *California Safe Care Standard* campaign also redefined its meaning of workplace violence to the same description that OSHA uses.

What makes OSHA's definition so great is that it not only includes both verbal and physical violence, but it also acknowledges actions that cause emotional and mental distress. The plan uses this definition and focuses on being all-inclusive, honoring the rights of healthcare workers, patients, visitors, and other hospital clients.

Mandatory Training as Defined by the SB 1299

The standards enforced by this bill make it necessary for workers to have appropriate training, much like the

---

[15] https://www.osha.gov/workplace-violence

Assembly Bill (AB 508). The Senate bill makes it mandatory for a workplace in the healthcare industry to include:

- **A violence prevention plan.** This should be specially designed to keep their healthcare professionals safe from violence and bullying.
- **Healthcare professionals who are in direct contact with special or dangerous patients should receive formal training.** Unlike AB 508, it mandates the need for one to have educational credits to know how to handle them.
- **Healthcare workers should know how to seek help.** They need to know how to respond to requests for assistance and prevent violence from happening to them or others around them.
- **Hospital healthcare professionals should know how to identify incidences of violence.** They also have to be taught how to:
  o Identify that a situation is violent
  o Know how and when to seek assistance
  o When they should respond to the violence themselves
- **Workplace violence prevention training should teach healthcare employees how to report a violent incident to law enforcement agencies.** Poor filing practices can ruin the credibility of a case. Training should focus on the crucial details they need to focus on. These include:
  o Details that can relate to the attacker
  o The weapon used or their actions. This will encourage vigilance and introduce accountability in actions that will reduce

the chances of another violent crime from happening.

- **The training has to teach healthcare workers about the resources at their disposal if a violent incident occurs in the workplace.** These resources should also include tools for helping healthcare workers cope with the aftermath of violent incidents.
- **Healthcare employees have to know the potential risks they face in certain parts of the hospital**. For example, they may face threats when working near parking lots.
- **Hospitals are required to document every violent incident that occurred at the hospital's premises.** Documentation is also needed for violent incidents where there was no injury done to the victim.
- **SB 1299 makes it mandatory for hospitals to have security systems that include alarms, security personnel at the hospital premises, and emergency responses for active shooter situations at the hospital.** Hospitals must assess their security measures and make appropriate improvements where needed.
- **Proper protocols for security are needed at a hospital to ensure that there is a quick response.** Quick security responses can prevent a situation from turning violent and minimize the damage caused by an assailant.
- **Hospitals are also required to provide temporary employees with an orientation session on workplace violence prevention.** Employees have to know what measures to take

to prevent workplace violence, even if they are not permanent employees.

It's clear to see that Senate Bill 1299 builds upon and adds more to the requirements for mandatory training that were introduced in Assembly Bill 508. What's unfortunate is that even though these bills were passed in 2014 and 1993, there are few hospitals and organizations that are compliant with them.

With shrinking budgets, one of the first areas that hospitals tend to cut corners on is their training sessions. It is a significant contributor to why workplace violence is so prevalent in the healthcare industry.

Having an Effective Workplace Violence Prevention Plan (WVPP)

According to OSHA, offices should have a workplace violence prevention plan (WVPP) that meets the following needs:

- Decreases the chances of injury, loss of life, or more because of workplace violence.
- Reduce the overall costs of indirect and direct workplace violence.
- Improve the perception of employees regarding their workplace and improve their sense of well-being, safety, and security at work.

What Should an Effective Workplace Violence Prevention Plan Cover?

When you are beginning to make a workplace violence prevention plan (WVPP), you need to ensure that your plan will cover the following core areas and tools:

- A written policy for the implementation and monitoring of the workplace violence prevention program
- Assigning responsibility relating to the WVPP to a selected team that will function in the company
- Adoption of disciplinary procedures that are fair and consistent in providing punishment for those committing workplace violence
- Development of methods through which the WVPP will provide information and communicate with all employees(future and present)
- Develop procedures that will assess the overall potential for violence through methods like peer reviews, inspections for workplace violence, and employee surveys.
- Development of appropriate strategies for control and prevention of workplace violence
- Documenting and providing regular training to all managers and employees
- Stringent procedures will be relied upon to conduct thorough investigations of all incidents of workplace violence.
- Providing appropriate support without discriminating against witnesses or victims of workplace violence
- A systematic methodology to evaluate practices and revise the workplace violence prevention program as needed.

Developing a Team for the Workplace Violence Prevention Program

Many successful violence prevention programs start with a collaborative group. This group is responsible for handling all reports of incidents. This group should also have the capacity to actively assess the company's ability to deal with the incidents they have identified.

Moreover, the group should have suggestions to strengthen their ability to provide appropriate responses to the significant issue. Members of this group should be a mix of management and labor-based individuals and should be picked from the following groups:

- Safety Team
- Health and Medical Team
- Security
- Law Enforcement
- Human Resource

Even if the members of this team are not directly responsible for handling the incidents, they can work as consultants to provide input, feedback, and insight into various areas that the workplace violence prevention program needs to improve.

Identifying Major Risk Factors
It is also necessary to identify the significant risk factors that a person faces that can contribute to instances of workplace violence. These factors include the following:

- Do the employees have direct contact with individuals from the public?
- Do they handle any vital functions, such as the exchange of money?
- Is there any illegal activity occurring near or on the work premises, such as selling drugs?
- Is the workplace primarily mobile in nature?
- Is exposure to an unstable or volatile person likely to happen?

- Do any of the employees work alone, or do they work in a small team?
- Do the employees occasionally choose to work late at night or during the early morning hours?
- Do employees have to work in areas with high crime rates?
- Do the employees handle valuable property or have visibly valuable possessions?
- Do the employees have the power to control the benefits, well-being, or freedom of others who work with them?

By assessing all these areas, it is possible to identify the risk that one can face. The workplace violence prevention program can have appropriate measures that effectively protect one from the risks they face due to the factors mentioned above.

Developing Preventative Control Strategies
Once the risks involved have been identified, it is time to develop appropriate control strategies that will be crucial to preventing workplace violence. The strategies should not only be thorough but may also include the following:

- Screening with the help of a thorough background check to identify the risk with potential employees that may have a history of violence
- Use appropriate drug tests for current and new employees periodically
- Provide access to an Employee Assistance Program with complete confidentiality to help employees overcome issues such as substance abuse and financial, emotional, and marital problems – a list of appropriate community-based resources can also be offered.

- Training for individuals who are responsible for handling incidents as well as helping them take appropriate responses for the incident that is brought to light
- Prompt investigation of all incidents of workplace violence
- Ensure proper communication and understanding of the policy for workplace violence prevention that applies to all the employees, the managers, and even the visitors
- Have a system that uses appropriate panic alarms or other forms of electronic devices that can be used to alert one to potential danger caused by an active workplace violence incident
- Have appropriate physical searches or use metal detectors to identify any guns, knives, or weapons on another person
- Make use of cameras and a closed-circuit system in the right locations to improve security on office premises
- Restrict access to areas with the help of key cards to prevent customers from accessing private, employee-only areas
- Have a sign-in system for all visitors and offer identification badges before allowing them access to the office premises
- Install curved mirrors in intersections in hallways or other areas to prevent blind spots
- Have bright lighting on the interior and exterior of a building, including on the parking areas, footpaths, and more
- Identify and replace any broken locks, fences, windows, or gates to improve security

- Ensure all vehicles are kept locked on the premises
- Remove the use of all items that can potentially be used as a weapon
- Provide employees with escorts to walk them to their cars at night or if situated in a high crime area
- Device a buddy system or offer disciplinary counseling for troubled employees

By developing these strategies, healthcare institutions can effectively tackle a large number of workplace violence issues in a healthy and appropriate manner.

Education of the Team
Once the program is developed, time must be spent educating the team about the policies. By paying close attention to this factor, one can also reduce the instances of workplace violence. The team's education has to be done in two parts: for the employees and the managers.

Employees
The employees need to be taught about the workplace violence prevention program in the following manner:

- A detailed explanation of the "zero tolerance "policy being implemented to prevent workplace violence.
- The requirements for as well as the procedures that they can use to report any incidents
- Outlining ways that one can prevent and diffuse volatile situations and handle aggressive behavior
- Deal safely with hostile persons and what they should do in such situations.
- Manage anger holistically with the help of the right coping mechanisms
- Learn vital skills and techniques to resolve conflicts peacefully and appropriately

- Techniques for effective stress management and training to ensure employee wellness
- The security procedures for various scenarios of violence in the workplace
- The personal security measures that one can adopt in instances of violence in the workplace
- Access to employee assistance programs and other similar options available for employees in the company to resolve conflicts

The Managers

Managers not only have to be trained to know the points mentioned above, but their training needs to go one step further. They also have to focus on the following:

- Identify how to encourage the employees to report workplace violence incidents effectively, especially when they are feeling threatened by another person, either inside or outside of the organization
- Improve their skills to learn how to behave supportively and compassionately towards all employees who are reporting incidents.
- Develop vital skills to implement disciplinary actions against the people who are found to be causing workplace incidents.
- Develop basic skills to handle crisis situations in the workplace effectively.
- Know the basic skills and emergency procedures for life-threatening or crisis situations in the workplace.
- Ensure that screening in pre-employment is done appropriately, even when handling references.

The Investigation Process of Threats

An investigation should be done thoroughly for all threats or actual incidents of harassment and workplace violence.

Never allow a victim to confront their aggressor; it can be potentially harmful to the well-being of both parties. At most, the investigation should involve a detailed review in the following areas with the help of a mediation team:

- Name of the person making the threat
  - Their relationship with the victim and the company
  - Their appearance
  - Their mental and emotional condition
- Name of the victim or the potential victim
  - Their relationship with the victim and the company
  - Their appearance
  - Their mental and emotional condition
- Where and when did the incident happen?
  - What happened right after the incident?
  - How was the incident brought to an end?
- The language explicitly used to make the threat.
- If any kind of physical action was taken – this will substantiate the claim or solidify the intention that one is going to take further action on the threat they made
- Names of anyone else who was directly or indirectly involved
  - Any kind of action that they took
- Names of any witnesses
- Names of supervisory staff (if they were involved)
  - What kind of response did they take
- What was the reason for the incident?
  - Any signs that were overlooked or history of violence and more
- The extent of the damage
  - Will the authorities have to be involved?

- o Is their physical and verbal abuse?
- o Can mediation help?

These steps can ensure a thorough investigation and will make sure that your workforce feels safer. It's also a crucial step to take when considering a solution to the problem.

What to do if there is a Real Threat

If there is a credible threat or incident of violence, you can then start to implement the following:

- Consequences after the incident
  - o What will happen to the person making the threats?
  - o What will happen to the employees who were victimized or directly involved in the scenario?
- Report the incident to the law enforcement authorities
  - o Help them with their legal proceedings
  - o Provide accurate information to law enforcement agencies, media outlets, or other agencies.
- Use an emergency code to launch the protocol that one must take to secure all the work areas where the incident occurred.
- Take active measures to account for the well-being of all the employees and ensure that other people in the area are physically safe from any other harm.
- Make sure that another work area is not short-staffed when others are busy assisting the victim or helping to secure the perimeters.
- Provide a confidential one-on-one debriefing of the incident to the victims, the witnesses, and other employees affected by it.

Treatment for the Victims

While it is important to report, investigate, and promptly respond to all incidents of workplace violence, having a response to deal with the aftermath of the incident is necessary. You should have a comprehensive treatment plan available for the victims and the other employees affected by the incident.

Right after an incident, the victims, witnesses, or even first responders from your team may experience:

- Emotional trauma (Short term or long-term)
- Fear or hesitancy about going back to work
- Changes in behavior and their relationships with their co-workers or their family
- Intense feelings of guilt
- Powerlessness or helplessness

The plan should be vital to aiding in the recovery and assisting the employee in moving forward from the ordeal. These steps should also be focused on helping the victim or any other people involved recover and move on from the incident in a healthy manner.

Regular Evaluation of the Workplace Violence Prevention Plan (WVPP)

Once you have the workplace violence prevention plan in place, you should evaluate and revise it regularly, mainly if a workplace incident has occurred. This ensures that there are no areas that are being left out in your workplace violence prevention plan.

The process of evaluation should be done with the help of knowledgeable employees, such as the ones who are on the response team for these threats. With their help, you can do the following:

- Run an in-depth audit to determine which components of the program are currently active successfully
- Measure the improvement brought about with the help of the program
  - This should be based on the lowered frequency and the severity of incidents of workplace violence.
- Conduct an employee satisfaction survey and review the overall results
- Identify the areas where there is room for improvement
  - Develop effective strategies to improve this area
- Train, educate, and implement the changes that are being made to the program

By having a continually updated plan, you can ensure that you don't experience workplace violence through ignorance or by failure to have a proper plan in place. Being proactive in this area will play a massive role in ensuring that the workplace stays safe and the lives of all the employees and customers are not at risk.

Why Nurses Face Violence and Bullying in the Workplace

Nursing is widely regarded as one of the most respected professions, yet workplace violence and bullying remain persistent problems. Many nurses find themselves subjected to these troubling experiences, but why is this so common in a field dedicated to care and healing?

The causes are varied and often overlooked. Below are some of the key factors contributing to the violence and bullying nurses face in their workplaces.

Staff Shortage

The ongoing nurse shortage in the U.S. healthcare system has created a stressful environment for many nurses. With fewer staff members available, nurses are often pushed to their limits, leading to a high-stress atmosphere that fosters bullying and violence. The lack of adequate staffing means that many nurses work long hours with little to no breaks, often getting just a few minutes to rest during their shifts. The constant pressure is not only physically exhausting but also mentally draining. Over time, it wears down their resilience and ability to cope.

According to a research finding, when nurses are fatigued, their ability to perform their duties can be affected.[16] Mistakes become more likely, putting them at risk of frustration or aggression from patients, their families, or

---

[16] Stimpfel, A. W., & Aiken, L. H. (2013). Hospital staff nurses' shift length associated with safety and quality of care. Journal of nursing care quality, 28(2), 122–129. https://doi.org/10.1097/NCQ.0b013e3182725f09

even colleagues. Physical and verbal abuse from patients or their attendants is not uncommon. In some cases, nurses are blamed for errors that result from an overwhelming workload, further fueling workplace tension.

Bullying from Charge Nurses

Benner's stages of clinical competence describe how nurses develop skills and gain experience over time. These stages are:

1. **Novice:** Beginners with no experience who rely on rules and guidelines to perform tasks.
2. **Advanced Beginner:** Nurses with some experience who can identify recurring situations but still need support.
3. **Competent:** Nurses with two to three years of experience who can plan and manage patient care efficiently.
4. **Proficient:** Nurses who have a deeper understanding of patient care and can quickly assess situations.
5. **Expert:** Highly experienced nurses who no longer rely on rules and can provide intuitive and skillful care.

Charge nurses are RNs who are given additional responsibilities, such as overseeing other nurses, managing the unit, and ensuring smooth patient care. They act as the point of contact for both the nursing staff and administration. A charge nurse should ideally be at the **Proficient** or **Competent** stage. However, some nurses are assigned the role of charge nurse without having sufficient experience, sometimes with less than six months or a year in the field. This lack of experience can make them uncomfortable, especially when dealing with more seasoned travel or registry nurses who bring years of expertise.

In these situations, less experienced charge nurses may feel inadequate, leading to insecurity. As a result, they may develop unfair attitudes towards more experienced R.N.s, such as shortening break times and increasing workload unnecessarily.

Nursing can sometimes feel like a battlefield, not because of the physical demands but due to the mental toll caused by bullying within the profession. It's often compared to gangbangers — nurses may not be physically harming each other, but the emotional and psychological strain inflicted through bullying is just as damaging.

This toxic environment has led many nurses to take stress leave, and some have even left the profession altogether. In extreme cases, the mental strain has driven some nurses to lash out at their colleagues, further worsening the workplace atmosphere. According to research, emotional strain can become the trigger point for such incivility in the workplace.[17] Unfortunately, such instances are far more common in nursing than in any other profession.

Nurses dedicate their lives to caring for patients, but in reality, many are suffering silently, becoming "walking patients" themselves, struggling under the weight of the mental stress brought on by bullying.

In many cases, the charge nurses even end up issuing DNR/DNS (do not return/do not send) orders for travel nurses because of their discomfort rather than legitimate concerns. This practice can create tension in the workplace and may unfairly penalize competent nurses.

---

[17] Loh, Jennifer M I, and Abu Saleh. "Lashing out: emotional exhaustion triggers retaliatory incivility in the workplace." Heliyon vol. 8,1 e08694. 30 Dec. 2021, doi:10.1016/j.heliyon.2021.e08694

Racism

Racism in the nursing field is a pressing issue, with many nurses experiencing or witnessing it firsthand, not just from patients but from colleagues as well. According to a survey of 900 nurses, 60% reported experiencing or observing racist behavior from their co-workers. However, fewer than 1 in 4 actually reported these incidents, often fearing that their concerns would not be taken seriously by human resources, administrators, or even their union leaders. Over half of those who did report racist incidents found that it damaged their relationships with supervisors and colleagues.[18]

There is a disturbing culture in some hospitals where certain racial or ethnic groups are referred to as the "MAFIA" due to their hostile treatment of other cultures. This type of bullying and exclusion leads to a toxic work environment, causing mental strain and pushing many nurses to leave the profession. The racial breakdown of the nursing workforce in 2022 shows:

- 80% of registered nurses are White
- 7.4% are Asian
- 6.3% are Black
- 2.5% identify as more than one race
- 6.9% of nurses report their ethnicity as Hispanic[19]

The imbalance in representation creates an environment where minority nurses often feel isolated or marginalized. Many nurses of color report feeling unsupported, and they hesitate to speak up about the discrimination they face, knowing it could lead to retaliation or strained relationships.

---

[18] https://www.statnews.com/2023/05/31/nursing-racism-survey/
[19] https://www.aacnnursing.org/news-data/fact-sheets/nursing-workforce-fact-sheet

Racism in the workplace, especially when left unchecked, is not just a personal issue; it weakens the entire healthcare system by driving qualified and dedicated professionals out of their careers. It's important to address these concerns directly to create a more inclusive and respectful work environment for all nurses.

Aggravated Patients or Attendants

Patients who are experiencing pain and suffering may take their frustration out on the hospital staff. A lot of registered nurses work with people who are not emotionally stable. These patients might also act out physically and violently.

Healthcare workers are also bound to come in close physical contact with them, so they are vulnerable to physical attacks and other abuse from them. Even if nurses try to be compassionate, they can get abused for their empathy.

The relatives of patients can also inflict violence and cause abuse against registered nurses. Relatives and family members may feel stressed out, overburdened, or upset and might lash out at the nurses.

A shortage of hospital staff can also result in worried family members, who might take out their anger on the team that is already present. Proper know-how is necessary to de-escalate the situation successfully.

Overcrowding in hospitals is also another reason why violence against healthcare workers is so widespread. Even though the nurses are not to blame in this case, the patients may not see it that way.

Frustrated at being packed into a small building for hours or days may cause them to take out their anger and frustrations on the nurses.

Attitude Problems

One of the often overlooked reasons for violence or bullying against nurses is their attitude, which is more times than not shaped by the high-stress nature of their job. Long hours, exhausting work, and witnessing suffering and death day after day can take a serious toll on a nurse's mental and emotional state.

Nurses also deal with difficult supervisors, co-workers, and patients while often feeling underappreciated by doctors, patients, and their families. The combination of pressures leads to burnout, causing some nurses to become irritable or detached in their interactions.

When a nurse is exhausted and emotionally drained, it may become harder to maintain a calm and friendly demeanor. The stress and fatigue may affect the way they communicate, making them seem unapproachable or short-tempered. While the nurse may be struggling internally, the other party — whether a patient, family member or colleague — might not see this. Instead, they may misinterpret the nurse's behavior as dismissive or uncaring, which can lead to frustration and, in some cases, bullying or outright aggression toward the nurse.

In healthcare settings, the stakes are already high. Misunderstandings or tension between nurses and others can escalate quickly, especially when emotions are already running high due to illness, loss, or fear. Nurses, being on the frontlines, often bear the brunt of this, even when their own attitude is shaped by the immense pressure they face daily.

Lack of Training

Lack of early training is a major reason why healthcare workers face bullying and violence at work. Nursing students, in particular, are often unprepared to handle such situations, which can make them more vulnerable. Training in recognizing the signs of violence and preventing bullying should be mandatory for all healthcare workers, especially those in nursing. This training should begin well before clinical rotations, giving students the tools to navigate the challenges of a hospital environment.

Nursing students have to face difficult situations when they are paired with experienced nurses during their clinical training. Without proper training in dealing with workplace bullying and violence, these students may find themselves at the mercy of senior nurses who, due to stress or their own experiences, can be unkind or even cruel. The mistreatment affects their learning and can dampen their progress in the nursing program. Instead of gaining valuable experience, students may be left feeling discouraged or demoralized.

Some wonder if bullying starts in nursing schools. The behavior some students face during their training might carry over into their professional lives, leading to a cycle of bullying in healthcare. When students experience negative treatment early on, they may internalize it, and this behavior can seep into the workplace as they move into their careers.

Do Not Return (DNR) – What it Means

We have mentioned briefly in earlier chapters that doctors, supervisors, or charge nurses can give a DNR (Do Not Return) notice to co-workers, particularly registry or travel nurses, that they do not like. Many people are not aware of what a DNR is since it only affects a niche demographic in the healthcare industry.

This is a significant reason why it is used so effectively to ruin the very livelihood of registry and travel nurses. However, it is essential to learn about this and to understand how it is actively misused to bring this trend to a stop.

What is a DNR (Do Not Return) Notice?
A DNR (Do Not Return) notice is also known as a DNS (Do Not Send) or a DNU (Do Not Use). It is a document that can be used to end a contract with a registry or travel nurse who is hired through a staffing agency.

DNRs are commonly used in the healthcare industry, particularly if hospitals are choosing to hire temporary nurses through the help of a staffing agency. The duration of the work period is determined when the contract is signed.

During this time period, nurses have to work according to the standards for quality as enforced by the hospital. Moreover, hospitals that are hiring through a staffing agency cannot terminate a contract as they see fit. They must work with the nurse for the duration of the contract, whether 6 weeks or 13 weeks.

However, if the nurse violates a hospital policy or fails to meet the quality standards of the hospital, despite repeated warnings, the hospital staff, often the charge nurse, can give the nurse in question a DNR. Given this aspect, in theory, and practice, termination through DNR should only be considered for severe offenses.

Unfortunately, hospitals can also rely on a DNR to terminate their contract early. To terminate their contract with the registry or travel nurse, the hospital has to blacklist that nurse with a DNR. In this way, the hospital will be spared from paying any kind of cancellation fee.

The hospital might be saving money in this case, but they are destroying the career of that nurse. A DNR goes one step further than simple termination, as it also works like a blacklisting option against the nurse.

This is a notice that goes on the permanent work record of the nurse. It conclusively shows that the hospital will not work with a particular nurse again, which can cause the nurse to face a lot of backlash in the healthcare industry.

Bullying Through DNR

One of the major issues is that the DNR is misused on such a large scale. Even more worrying is how quick hospitals, doctors, and charge nurses are at handing out DNR notices to nurses that they do not like. It might seem like it is something of little consequence to them, but a DNR can spell disaster for these registry and travel nurses.

Other forms of bullying that registry and travel nurses can feel because of a DNR are:

- **Leaves Them Vulnerable to Bullying** – Certain charge nurses can threaten to give a DNR to a nurse with a spotless record unless they do what they say. In such cases, either they will have to deal with the harassment and backlash of a DNR. They are also more likely to have their work abilities hampered. This causes an abusive cycle in which colleagues doubt the affected nurses' credibility, and the stress from that doubt prevents these nurses from working effectively.

- **Ruins Future Employment Chances** – Once a nurse gets a DNR on their permanent record, it can ruin their chances of finding future employment elsewhere. It is something that goes on the permanent record of a registry or travel nurse. This means that when they are being hired by a different hospital, they will see the DNR notice. It can also prompt the hospital to skip over the nurse.

- **Defamation of Their Character** – It causes the nurse to face extreme defamation, which may or may not be valid. There is a very high possibility that a terminated nurse did nothing wrong but had to deal with the consequences of the DNR.

- **Discrimination at the Workplace** – Even when the nurse does acquire any employment elsewhere, they may face discrimination from their colleagues because of the DNR on their record of accomplishments. These nurses may have the credibility of their work frequently questioned by other healthcare workers.

- **Harms Their Mental Health** – Nurses with a DNR are usually met with suspicion, constant surveillance, and doubt at a new workplace. This can make them feel anxious that they may have to undergo a similar blacklisting process at their current workplace. This can cause stress and depression and will gravely harm their mental health and their emotional well-being.

- **Destroys Their Career** – Many registry and travel nurses may also be forced to look into different career options because of the difficulty of finding one in healthcare. Nurses with a DNR will find it extremely difficult to work successfully. Given the many years it takes for one to become a nurse, a DNR can be a death sentence to the career of a registry or a travel nurse. They may never be able to find employment in another hospital because of it, which further aggravates the issue of nurse shortage discussed in the previous chapters.

It should be remembered that in a majority of the DNR cases, the registry or travel nurse is someone who did not do anything wrong. Wrongfully getting a DNR notice can be extremely harmful to a registry and travel nurse, not just emotionally, mentally, and physically, but also financially. Here are just a few examples of unfair use of DNR/DNS notices:

- A nurse forgot to document vital signs. Even if they did, a charge nurse should have reminded them, especially during the initial adjustment period.
- A travel nurse was using their cellphone to order food, while others were using theirs to show off travel photos or use social media. Still, the simple task becomes grounds for a DNR, even though it does not interfere with patient care.
- A travel nurse decided not to renew their contract.
- A patient's colostomy bag was full, and it was used as grounds for action.
- A registry nurse discharged a patient per the doctor's orders, but the patient didn't receive their scheduled C.T. scan.

- A nurse asked for help when overwhelmed but was seen by the charge nurse as needy or slow.
- A patient's family complained, even though the nurse was helpful and worked well with the rest of the team.
- A nurse, initially scheduled for one unit, was reassigned to another. After expressing that their original assignment was different, they were placed on DNR/DNS.
- The nurse didn't "fit in" with the culture of the unit or team.
- The nurse spoke their native language around English-speaking colleagues.

Real-Life Accounts of Unfair DNR/DNS
The above were just examples; below are some real-life cases where travel and registry nurses were given DNR/DNS notices on petty issues:

1. A veteran nurse with a career of 10 years with great written evaluations and positive verbal accolades from patients and regular staff once gave a verbal report to an incoming nurse. The veteran nurse soon learned from her nursing registry agency that she was labeled DNR/DNS because the incoming nurse reported that a patient's colostomy bag had not been changed.
2. A traveling RN who was at the end of his traveling contract was offered an extension. However, he declined the extension, which led to him being labeled a DNR/DNS by the hospital.
3. An out-of-state traveling nurse was being trained in computer charting for electronic medical records (EMR). The following day, the hospital asked her to

train another travel nurse on the EMR. The next day, her agency informed her that she had been labeled DNR/DNS because of her "poor" computer documentation when she had only been in that hospital for 3 days. Unfortunately, she had to pack up and return to her state.

4. One registry nurse who could execute multiple roles (e.g., ER, ICU, House Supervisor) was personally requested by a hospital's director. On one shift, this talented nurse had to bring a patient to MRI after 06:00. When the nurse returned from the MRI, the new charge nurse stated that they had to clean his remaining ICU patients. However, the agency informed him that he became DNR/DNS because his patient was "dirty."

5. A nurse became a DNR/DNS because the doctor gave discharge instructions despite the patient having a pending CT scan. The patient was discharged without a CT scan. The nurse in question received termination while the doctor continued working without facing any issues.

The worst part about these unfair and baseless DNR/DNS notices is that not every registry or travel nurse is aware of what to do in such cases. Luckily, we're going to be taking a closer look at this aspect.

Got DNR'd? Here's What You Can Do

No matter what situation you are in, always know that you have rights as a professional and as a citizen. The same applies to registry and travel nurses. Even when faced with a DNR, you have certain rights that you can exercise in this case.

Unfortunately, most nurses are usually too overwhelmed by the immediate effects of a DNR to consider this aspect. However, if you have been wrongfully terminated with the use of a DNR, you have the right to contest it.

Additionally, many hospitals often do not give a reason for placing someone on DNR. Unless you actively reach out to them, few will provide more details about their decision. If you want to contest a DNR, you can do so in the following manner:

Ask the Agency to Evaluate the Case
When you are given a DNS, you can ask the staffing agency to evaluate it for you. Ask them to get more details and get to the nature of the complaints. Asking the agency to get involved on your behalf will ensure the following:

- In certain scenarios, the management may be more comfortable sharing details with them instead of with you
- The staffing agency will also understand when the hospital is trying to avoid cancellation fees for early termination.
- This is especially true if a travel or registry nurse has worked on assignments without any incident, and the

staffing agency is suddenly getting many complaints about the nurse.

- You will easily get a natural mediator for you and the hospital to evaluate the issue and get a satisfactory outcome.

Never assume that the staffing agency will not back you up. As registry and travel nurses, you are helping them earn money and are the biggest asset – if the agency does not protect its assets from misuse, it is not a good company.

Mediation Meeting

The normal protocol for any issues that arise is to have a mediation meeting. In this case, the doctor, charge nurse, administrator, or another person who has a professional, legitimate complaint should approach the staffing agency. By doing so, they have the opportunity to identify the issues and get them addressed properly.

Hospitals that provide no reason for a DNR usually do not understand the ramifications of their actions. By offering no explanation, they are damaging the working ability of competent nurses and shielding the nurses who need more training or counseling.

With a mediation meeting, all these issues can be brought to light. Then, the travel nurse should be given opportunities for coaching and counseling to improve their performance and to fix the issues pointed out. With mediation meetings, both parties can air out the issues in the workplace without having to resort to any untoward actions.

Make Sure There Was No Serious Infraction

In some cases, an investigation into a DNR is needed to make sure that there was no severe infraction of the professional laws. Remember that a DNR is mainly meant to deal with nurses who may pose a threat to their patients.

It is also for nurses who did not meet the rules and regulations of the hospital despite getting repeated warnings. Actions that can fall within this category can include the following:

- Drinking while on the job
- Using drugs illegally
- Stealing medication from patients
- Neglecting patients
- Bullying or harassing co-workers
- Failing to work within the hospital's rules and regulations
- Placing others around them in danger because of their carelessness

If a nurse's actions do not fall into any of the categories mentioned above, they do not qualify to have a DNR used against them. If the nurse is genuinely at fault, then the agency has to take appropriate action and train the nurse, offer employee support systems, or more to fix the issue at hand.

Look for Missing Details and Paperwork
A majority of the DNR cases that are issued are usually done so over small, petty issues. Moreover, it can also be when the hospital does not want to deal with the penalty of ending the contract early. Given the laws for wrongful termination, hospitals cannot terminate employees without any appropriate documentation about the issues.

These include the following:

- Recorded narratives from witnesses:

- o The names of the witnesses
  - o The time and date
- Workplace evidence and records that include:
  - o Computer logins
  - o Time in and time out
  - o Station assignments
  - o Patient assignments

Documentation is necessary to back up all the complaints that the hospital administration is making. If the complaints have no documentation narrative, it can be seen that the DNR was issued wrongfully. In this case, they might be liable for a lawsuit.

If you have done the steps mentioned above and no clear issues have popped up, you can then choose to take legal action.

Wrongful Termination Lawsuit

In many cases, a DNR may also be given when a change of management happens. In this case, it can be surprising to see that a nurse who has a spotless profile and career history with a hospital is now suddenly being placed on DNR.

In such scenarios, a hospital can be liable for a wrongful termination lawsuit from the travel or registry nurse. A wrongful termination lawsuit can be filed against the hospital administration if they meet the following requirements:

- When a DNR is handed out for no valid reason
- A reason to suggest that the hospital deliberately opted for the DNR at the first mistake without taking other precautionary measures
- Lack of documentation that supports the hospital's complaints against the nurse.

- Refusal to mediate and discuss the issue properly with the nurse

Moreover, it is not just the hospital that can be sued; the staffing agency can also be sued. Appropriate evidence must be provided to ensure that the staffing agency did everything in its power to support and represent the nurse given a DNR.

By making sure that you pay attention to these factors, you can easily exercise your rights. It also gives you more confidence to know that when faced with a DNR, it doesn't mean that your career has ended. Yes, things are tough, but there is always a solution, and you are well within your rights to practice the steps outlined in this area.

DNR Mitigation and Prevention – Strategies to Follow

Although nurses have certain rights they can exercise when faced with a DNR or DNS notice, the current system often leaves travel and registry nurses at a disadvantage. This is a critical issue that calls for change. More strategies focused on preventing these unfair practices and resolving conflicts must be implemented within the healthcare sector.

These steps are essential not only for ensuring job security for nurses but also for addressing the ongoing nurse shortage. Creating a more stable, supportive, and fair work environment will also promote the well-being of both staff and patients.

That said, here are some DNR mitigation and prevention strategies that can be implemented in hospitals:

Introduction of a Feedback Form

The introduction of a feedback form for travel and registry nurses is an important step in improving workplace conditions. The form is developed specifically for travel and registry nurses, allowing them to evaluate their experience at the hospital. More importantly, managers and directors can assess how well their staff treats temporary nurses and how they can create a more supportive environment by using the insights nurses have documented.

Here's the form designed by Empirical Safety Training:

Empirical Safety Training

Registry Nurse Experience Feedback

Employee Information			
Name		**Shift**	
Date		**Department**	

Quality Ratings					
	1 Poor	2 Fair	3 Average	4 Good	5 Excellent
How was your staffing Office experience?	☐	☐	☐	☐	☐
Comments					
How were you greeted upon your arrival at your assigned unit?	☐	☐	☐	☐	☐
Comments					
How comprehensive was your shift report?	☐	☐	☐	☐	☐
Comments					
How was your interaction with the staff during your shift on the assigned unit?	☐	☐	☐	☐	☐
Comments					
How resourceful were the staff members in the unit?	☐	☐	☐	☐	☐
Comments					
Did you receive an orientation to your assigned unit, including a	☐	☐	☐	☐	☐

crash cart, fire alarms/ extinguisher, and exit locations?					
Comments					
Do you feel you received adequate computer training?	☐	☐	☐	☐	☐
Comments					
Were you offered a break and lunch in a timely fashion?	☐	☐	☐	☐	☐
Comments					
Overall, how would you rate your registry experience?	☐	☐	☐	☐	☐
Comments					

Evaluation
ADDITIONAL COMMENTS

One of the key benefits of the feedback form is that it provides an opportunity for nurses to document any unfair treatment they may have experienced during their tenure. If unfair DNR/DNS decisions were made, this form allows the affected nurse to provide details, which can be used to investigate and address these concerns.

The feedback form will also help identify any instances of workplace bullying, especially from charge nurses or other senior staff. By gathering this information, hospital management can better understand where gaps in communication, training, or support may exist and take steps to improve them. This form encourages transparency and accountability, which are essential for building a healthier and more respectful work environment for all staff.

Here, I would like to thank Nikki Foots, RN. Her input has been truly valuable in putting together the Registry Feedback Form.

Handling Feedback and DNR Review Process

After the submission of the feedback form, it is crucial for the supervisor or manager to thoroughly review the comments. This includes carefully examining any issues raised by travel or registry nurses at the end of their tenure or after receiving a DNR notice. The goal is to identify where things may have gone wrong and whether any unfair treatment or bullying occurred, especially from the charge nurse or other staff members. If such behavior is found, immediate action must be taken to address it.

For nurses issued a DNR, the process doesn't end there. After 90 days, the nurse should be called back for a re-evaluation meeting. In this meeting, the supervisor or manager should hear the nurse's side of the story and also invite the person who issued the DNR. The goal is to resolve any conflicts and understand what led to the DNR being issued. If it is determined that the DNR was unjustified, it should be canceled, and disciplinary action should be taken against those responsible. This sends a message that unfair practices will not be tolerated.

To prevent in-hospital bullying and the misuse of DNR notices, managers should take the following steps:

- **Encourage open communication:** Create a work environment where staff feel comfortable voicing concerns without fear of retaliation.
- **Provide anti-bullying training:** All staff, especially those in leadership roles, should undergo training to recognize and prevent bullying.
- **Monitor charge nurse behavior:** Ensure that charge nurses treat all staff fairly, especially travel and registry nurses who may feel more vulnerable.
- **Implement clear reporting procedures:** Make it easy for nurses to report bullying or unfair treatment, and ensure these reports are handled promptly.
- **Hold staff accountable:** When bullying or unfair treatment is confirmed, enforce strict disciplinary actions to deter future incidents.
- **Conduct regular reviews:** Regularly evaluate staff interactions and address any recurring issues before they escalate.

Implementing these steps will help hospitals retain skilled nurses and ensure that DNR notices aren't issued unfairly.

Active Shooter Situations – How to Deal with Them

Did you know that hospitals now include active shooters in their emergency drills for disasters? From 2000 to date, there have been a total of 154 shootings in 148 hospitals.[20]

So, we're going to take a closer look at them here. An active shooter is a person who is a mass murderer. They are actively attempting to kill people in a populated area without or with a weapon (usually a firearm). The United States Department of Homeland Security has its definition of an active shooter.

According to them, an active shooter is *"An individual actively engaged in killing or attempting to kill people in a confined and populated area; in most cases, active shooters use firearms, and there is no pattern or method to their selection of victims."* It's common for active shooter situations to take place in schools, banks, hospitals, workplaces, and even houses of worship.

Active shooter situations are perilous because there is no specific target for the shooters in this case. The lack of a specific target automatically means that every person present in the space is a target and is in danger of being shot or harmed by the shooter.

An active shooter may continue shooting and causing harm to people until they are subdued or until the authorities are there. That is why spaces like hospitals need to have the right security present on the premises at all times. If appropriate

---

[20] https://www.ncbi.nlm.nih.gov/books/NBK519067/

help is available, active shooter events can be controlled within 10 to 15 minutes. It is rare for them to extend hours.

The presence of security personnel at a hospital acts as a deterrent for violent incidents, and it also ensures that there will be a quick response to an active shooter situation. In this way, the active shooter can be apprehended by security personnel or law enforcement authorities before they're able to do much harm to the people who are present in that space.

According to a report released by the FBI, the following are the success rates and expected outcomes for control of active shooter scenarios:

- 56.3% through the suicide of the shooter
- 28.1% through force by security or police
- 13.1% through force by unarmed citizens

A large majority of active shooters choose to commit suicide after they are finished with the crime. Or, they are shot and killed or choose to surrender when a big confrontation with the police becomes unavoidable.

An active shooter situation can be traumatic for all the people who have experienced it. Therefore, it can be difficult for healthcare workers who were present during an active shooter situation to cope with the stress and trauma related to the event.

The good thing is that both AB 508 and SB 1299 make it mandatory for hospitals to educate their workers on what resources they have at their disposal to cope with the traumatic event. In this way, healthcare workers can collectively work on improving their mental health so that they can move forward from the traumatic event.

Moreover, OSHA also updated its safety field Rule 3148 for healthcare, *Guidelines for Preventing Workplace Violence for Healthcare and Social Service Workers*. They made it mandatory for every healthcare facility to include appropriate solution management for such scenarios.

Based on this, most hospitals have actively developed codes that they can use for the scenario. The code will mean that people are aware of what's happening and don't run towards the sounds of the gunshot. Just announcing that it's a *'Code Grey'* should tell your team to call the emergency phone number and make their way to the emergency exits while helping as many people as possible.

What Do You Do in an Active Shooter Scenario?
In an active shooter scenario, you need to keep your cool and be diligent. Most of these scenarios last for 10 to 15 minutes, but they can cause a lot of casualties if care is not taken. If you ever find yourself in this scenario, the following is what you need to do to improve the chances of you and others to survive:

Step One - Evacuate
One of the first things that a person must do is take immediate action to evacuate the premises. To do this, you must do the following:

- Make sure that there is an exit near you.
- Leave all your belongings behind; you can always come back for them later.
- If there are law enforcement agents outside, approach them with your hands visible.
- If you are evacuating patients with special needs, inform the officials so that they can have the appropriate medical experts outside, too.

- Once outside, do not attempt to go back inside for others until the law enforcement officials allow you to do so. It may not be safe for you to do that.

Step Two - Hide

If you cannot make it to the emergency exits, or there isn't time to evacuate, you have to opt for step two in the following manner:

- Find a safe hiding spot that is not in the direct line of sight of the shooter.
- Look for places that also offer you protection but that won't trap you in a spot, such as the supply closet or the stairwell.
- Make sure to put your phone on silent, turn the lights off, and, if you can, place heavy furniture against the door to barricade it.
- If there's an exterior window, signal to the law enforcement agencies, but do not attempt to escape through that route until they let you know.

Step Three - Take Action

Step three is for scenarios when there's no other option but to attack the shooter. If you have to resort to step three, you can opt for the following:

- You can try to distract them, throw items at them, or even try to disarm them.
- Please note that this can be very dangerous and should be the last resort.
- In many cases, people have lost their lives while trying to subdue the shooter.

The U.S Department of Homeland Security mandates all these steps. These three steps are known to help save lives and take control of an active shooter situation.

Preparing for an Active Shooter Situation

However, apart from the steps mentioned above, hospitals also actively need to create an emergency plan for this. While you might have a code in place, it is also a good idea to practice how to make that emergency phone call.

Practicing this aspect beforehand will ensure that you or others can give the correct details to the authority. In this case, you have to make sure that when you answer the call, you have a set dialogue for communication.

This means that you make sure that you provide the following details:

- Where? – The location and address of the hospital
- How Many? – The total number of hostages and the shooters (that you know of)
- What? – Describe what has happened – whether you heard gunshots or saw someone waving a gun around.
- Details – Make sure to describe the weapon (if you can), whether it's a handgun or an assault rifle, etc.
- Don't End the Call – Even if you're unable to continue talking, leave the line clear so that the authorities can listen to the scenario.

Always make sure that every team member, especially new hires and interns, is aware of the emergency protocol, knows how to make a call to the authorities, and understands what to do in the event of an active shooter situation.

Additionally, if the hospital doesn't seem to have an emergency place, tell them that it's about time they made one. You can actively work with them to develop a tangible emergency plan that is easy to implement and will keep everyone safe.

Can DNRs Increase the Potential of Active Shooting?

As we previously discussed, getting a DNR notice can affect a nurse's mental and emotional well-being. Now, when placed in a crisis, many people typically recover by processing their loss.

On the other hand, there can be some who might feel resentful and upset with the life circumstances that they are in because of the DNR. For travel and registry nurses who received DNRs and rely on contracts with hospitals for work, the experience can be extremely traumatic, and they might want to get back at the hospital that did this to them.

The FBI studied cases of active shooters in the United States in 2023. According to their data, it was found that:

- Gender study revealed the composition of active shooters as follows:
    - 98% male
    - 1% female
    - 1% non-binary
- 48% of shooters have a known connection to the place of shooting or one of the victims[21]

In a study done by the U.S. Department of Justice, it was found that a large number of mass shooters *"frequently combined personal grievances (i.e., perceptions that they had been personally wronged) with political grievances (i.e.,*

---

[21]https://www.fbi.gov/file-repository/2023-active-shooter-report-062124.pdf/view

perceptions that a government entity or other political actor had committed an injustice)."

The report also highlighted that many individuals also resorted to violence because they felt:

- They had been discriminated against
- They were being treated unfairly
- They were being targeted by others

This may increase the desire of a person to get revenge on people who they feel have done them wrong. Additionally, there were other stress factors that made them feel this way. Most shooters experience the following major stressors:

- 49% experience financial strain
- 35% dealt with the job-related strain
- 29% had a conflict with their peers or friends
- 27% had marital or relationship problems
- 22% had alcohol or drug problems[22]

It's easy to see that when a person gets a DNR, they might experience all of the stressors mentioned above. For someone who feels trapped or like they have no other option available, this can be an extremely stressful situation to deal with.

While this doesn't mean that travel and registry nurses orchestrate mass shootings, it does highlight that a DNR, along with difficult life circumstances, can be a contributing factor to one's decision to do this.

---

[22] https://www.ojp.gov/pdffiles1/nij/250171.pdf

Conclusion

With the help of the information detailed in this book, I hope that nurses and hospitals can understand the dire situation of the healthcare industry and can make changes for the better. By adopting more compassion, understanding, and empathy towards each other, not only towards the patients, we can make a better work environment for everyone.

This book also raises awareness regarding the issues of DNR that travel and registry nurses face, as well as other issues, including active shooting incidents. It emphasizes the need for effective mediation programs and ethical solutions to create a safer, more cohesive work environment.

As part of this mission, I offer classes on Workplace Violence and Bullying Prevention as well as Active Shooter Training. I am actively working to get nursing schools to adopt these trainings for their students before they begin their clinical rotations so they are better equipped to handle these challenges. Students who complete the training under *Empirical Safety Training* will receive a certificate card that is valid for a year. Offering this training at a discounted rate ensures they enter the workforce ready and prepared to face these realities.

Even after graduation, nurses will still need to continue this training, but completing the course early can give them a head start in developing the skills necessary for a long, successful career. These trainings empower nurses to navigate the often difficult and stressful work environments they may encounter.

At *Empirical Safety Training*, we remain committed to conducting ongoing research to address workplace behavioral issues, boost team morale, and improve communication, all while adhering to OSHA guidelines. Together, we can work toward a better and safer healthcare system for all.

Thank you and best regards,

Made in the USA
Las Vegas, NV
18 March 2025

19785801R00049